FITDAMENTALS

**Fitness fundamentals that help REAL women
lose weight, have more energy,
and feel good in their own skin**

BY JENN VAZQUEZ

Publishing Services provided by Paper Raven Books
Printed in the United States of America
First Printing, 2017

ISBN 978-0-9991329-7-5

FREE GIFT

Thank you for buying this book!

As a free gift, please download the companion resources to jumpstart your fitness journey here:

www.fitdamentalsbook.com

TABLE OF CONTENTS

DEDICATION

This book is dedicated to my younger self and all the women who relate to her. May we find comfort and hope in each other's stories. Also, to my loving family who believed in me when I didn't believe in myself.

ACKNOWLEDGMENTS

It has truly taken a village to birth this book into the world. I have so many people to thank, it's hard to know where to start. Most likely, I have left someone out. If it's you, please forgive me and know that I value you.

Morgan and the Paper Raven Books Team, you have honestly been a pure joy to work with. This book would not have become a real thing without you. You have been so patient and encouraging. You validated my ideas and pushed me to get it into the world. I'm tearing up as I write this because I'm just so extremely grateful for you. I can honestly say that you have changed my life and I'm so blessed to know you and call you a friend.

My biz buddies who have challenged me and helped me grow, I would not have had the courage to take the first step, and every step after that, without you. Every mastermind group, every membership, every course, and every seminar has helped me learn and fine tune my message. If I met you through a group or event, please know you have made an impact in my life, and in this book. Special thanks to Tamsen Horton, Erin Smith, Coach Jennie, Holly Gillen, and Aldreama Harper who challenged me to think bigger during the year (plus) this book was being written.

All of my clients, both past and present, thank you for allowing me to be part of your life. Your time is precious and your health is priceless, so thank you for trusting me with two of your most valuable resources. It's a privilege and an honor I do not take for granted. A special thank you for smiling through the struggle, being open and honest, laughing at my bad jokes, and yelling "woo hoo" in class. (You know who you are!) I have the best job in the world and it's due to you. I only pray you have benefited as much as I have.

To my fellow fitness professionals and instructors, I am honored to be considered your peer. I have learned so much from you. I've admired this industry since I was a kid. To be part of it is a feeling I can't quite describe. It's nothing short of a dream come true and I thank you for making me feel welcome and valued in this strange new world. Special thanks to Nicole Esposito, Michele Park, Shari Littleton, and Kit Horton Caldicott for having faith in me and pushing me to be better at being me.

To my longtime friends and inner circle, you saw the evolution of Jenn and witnessed the events that became this book first hand. Thank you for not laughing at my crazy ideas (you actually encourage them!). Your confidence in me means the world. You know me better than most and you still stick around. My life is richer with you in it. Special thanks to Nitza, Stella, Vasthi, Liola, Annie, Michelle, Kathy, Cathy, Erin, Alan, and Laura.

To my siblings, aunts, uncles, cousins, and in-laws, I am truly a lucky lady to have such an amazing family. They say you can't pick your family, but I'd still pick you (even you, Mike). I am very blessed with so much love and support.

Mom, where do I even begin? You have always had unwavering confidence in me. You have stood by when I've made bad choices. You have been my biggest cheerleader. You are the most generous, kind, and loving person I know. Thank you for allowing me to make my own choices, for letting me fall, and for helping me get back up. But thank you most of all for believing that I can do anything.

Dad, thank you for giving me the example and inspiration to take the first step. I caught the marathon bug from you, and while I don't plan to catch up to you (I'll stick with two for now), I'm grateful for the all-in, over-the-top, stubborn genes you gave me. Thank you for making me feel like a princess and your favorite daughter, even if I am the problem child!

My boys, Josh and Isaiah, the greatest accomplishment of my life has been being your mom. You are both such sweet, kind young men. You give me pride and joy that nothing else compares to. Josh, my first born, you have been there by my side my entire adult life. Thank you for being so forgiving. I made many mistakes being a young mom, but somehow you turned out alright. Isaiah, my "baby boy," thank you for sharing your interests with me and allowing me into your creative world. I apologize for giving you my stubbornness and poor spelling skills. Thank you both for not being embarrassed by me (at least not out loud). You've always wanted to have me around and that is a blessing I value more than you know. Thanks for putting up with Nature

Walks, Game Nights, and Family Fun days! I love you both to infinity and beyond.

Dennis, the love of my life, my partner, my best friend, I honestly can't find the words to express my gratitude for your love and your ridiculous faith in me. You put up with my ever changing desires, and you encourage me to follow my dreams. You have supported me in every way through so many ups and downs. You are the most patient man I know, and I am honored to share this life with you. Thank you for loving me, believing in me, and seeing beauty in me when I didn't. Being your wife is the greatest joy of my life.

Finally, I could not end without thanking my Lord and Savior. I can do all things through Christ, and this book is living proof. When I am weak, You are Strong. My ultimate source of inspiration, determination, love, and joy. Thank you for leading my steps.

INTRODUCTION

You've tried almost every diet, workout plan, and supplement out there, but you're not losing weight, and you're still unhappy with your body. Can I be honest with you?

You've been lied to.

You've been told if you just cut calories and spend an hour on the elliptical five days a week, you'll get fit. You've been told if you drink smoothies and take expensive supplements, you'll drop pounds. But as a woman who struggled most of her life to get fit and finally found what really works, I can tell you that getting into shape is not as complicated as you've been led to believe. It can be simple, but you'll have to let go of the myths that are in all the glossy magazines and in your Instagram feed.

Let me give you a preview of some of the myth-busting things I want to talk with you about in this book:

- You need to drink *way* more water than you think you need to. That "8 glasses a day" thing is calculated for a 130-pound woman who doesn't drink coffee.
- All the diets that have you eliminating fruit or fat will not help you keep weight off in the long-term.
- Doing cardio every day may be good for your heart, but it will not change the shape of your body.
- Trouble spot specific exercises (like crunches for your abs) will not help you lose the fat you need to lose to zip up those skinny jeans.
- Stress could be the factor of your life that's causing you to yo-yo up and down, and keep putting the weight back on.

I have so much I want to share with you about how you can change your life, get into shape, and finally look and feel the way I know you want to. But first, let's talk about the *real* benefits of getting fit. If you want to skip right to the goodies, jump over to www.fitdamentalsbook.com for freebies to help you get started. Just make sure to come right back!

Empowerment. There is nothing quite like the feeling of pushing yourself physically and mentally past the point you thought possible. Doing things you've never done before (like a push up, for example) will give you a rush like you've never felt before. Increasing your strength (in body and mind) is one of the best things you can do for yourself, and it is the biggest boost in self-respect I've ever found. You'll be proud of what your body can do instead of focusing on what it cannot do.

Confidence. Along the same lines as empowerment, confidence will come as you make changes, stay consistent, and keep taking small steps toward the life you want. As you make positive, healthy choices, your resolve strengthens, and you begin to believe in yourself and your ability to finally do this once and for all. Each small step is a step toward a more confident, happy you. Conquering your workouts and your diet is a metaphor for life. When you have control over your body, you'll realize you have more control over other things. You'll walk taller, prouder, and finally be comfortable in your own skin. No more hating the reflection in the mirror. Very soon, you'll be looking in the mirror with amazement at how far you've come and just how amazing and beautiful you are. You just might even enjoy getting your picture taken instead of hiding from the camera.

You'll have improved health numbers, such as lower blood pressure, blood sugar, and positive comments from your doctor. You'll sleep better, have more energy, improve your mood, reduce your stress level, and learn to take care of yourself so you can take care of your loved ones. You might even have clearer skin, shinier hair, less bloating, and reduced joint pain. The benefits are numerous and priceless. It is worth the effort. You are worth the effort. Your loved ones deserve a happy, healthy you.

You will never waste time or money on another diet, gimmick, or desperate attempt to lose weight again! This is it! You will learn what you need to know to eat well, exercise, and start living a healthy life for good. You'll never fall for another weight loss fad again. You will be able to take what you learn and apply it to your life in your own way. You will learn guidelines instead of hard, fast rules.

You'll try new things. Not just new foods and new exercises, but you may decide to try a new hobby or activity. Maybe you'll take up running for the first time, or try skiing, zip lining, or some other physical activity you've been too insecure to try. The possibilities are endless.

Your dreams may become reality. Once you take control of your body, the life you've dreamed of is a small step away. You'll move on to improving your skills, knowledge, and relationships. Being happy and healthy is contagious. We are not happy just being satisfied with our physical selves—it's bigger than that. So much bigger. It's your life. It's your passions, dreams, and purpose. It starts with weight loss but, oh my dear friend, it's so much more. So much more.

My ultimate desire is for you to use your life, your energy, your health to make the world a better place for yourself, your loved ones, and the people around you. When you have vitality, health, and a clear mind, you can live up to the dreams and passions God has given you. You have many talents that are going unused because you are too tired, ill, or just plain scared to use them. When you are healthy and confident, you will finally be able to use them to their maximum potential and fulfill your purpose in this world.

Perhaps someone in your family or close circle needs to see you be successful to know they can take the first step too. We do not always know the impact we have on others. Let your life be an example to your loved ones. It is hard to take the first step, but if you stick with it, they will notice.

The legacy of self-hate, dieting, obesity, and insecurity ends here. It ends with you.

It's your time to shine. It's time for you to live each day with more vibrancy. Love more fully. Find more joy in each day. Shine your light for all to see.

Finally, the confidence boost that comes from taking care of yourself and doing things you thought were impossible is unlike anything I can describe. You will walk taller, hold your head up, smile bigger, and love your reflection in the mirror! You will have more energy to do the things you want to do with the people you love. You'll have more patience, kindness, and joy. You'll live with more love—love to others and love to yourself. Love, health, and joy will flow through you from the inside out.

Once you take care of yourself and start feeling great, results will come. It starts on the inside. Focus on how you FEEL, more than how you LOOK, and the results will take care of themselves. Poor health and being overweight is a symptom that something is off. When you start listening to your body and giving it things that it needs (and wants), your health, and your weight, will automatically improve. Yes, I know you want to look good, but it's way more than appearances. It's nice to look good, but it's more important to feel good and be healthy. Once you feel good and are healthier, weight loss is a very pleasant side effect. :)

Formula Overview

Here's how to create your own healthy life plan. Finally, the secret formula you've been waiting for! It has four parts. We will go into each part in detail later in the book. But if you're like me, you want the goods now. You want the overview and then you can decide if you want the details. Keep in mind that, in order to tweak your plan and create your own unique recipe for success, you will need to understand the details of each piece.

The basic formula looks like this: Water + Nutrition + Fitness + Rest = Results!

I told you it was simple and not incredibly surprising. The trick now is figuring out how to make each piece fit into your life. Do you have any idea where to start? No worries. I got you! We're going through this together and there is no rush. Take a deep breath and believe you can do this. You WILL do this.

The very first step is to identify which of these areas (water, nutrition, fitness, rest) to start with. One of these may be completely lacking or next to nothing (usually water or fitness), or it may be really poor (such as getting fewer than 6 hours of sleep or eating only take out/processed foods). Pick one. Just one! That's the magic of this approach. You do not have to turn your world upside down and change everything all at once. You will pick the one thing YOU know you need to improve.

Maybe you've been saying for months that you want to give up soda and drink more water. Then start there. Maybe you've been thinking about taking a walk at lunch. Do that. Maybe you know you're not getting enough sleep, burning the candle at both ends, waking up exhausted, and relying on caffeine to get through the day. Start by getting more sleep. Deep down, you know what you need to do. Trust yourself. Pick one thing and start there. If you're still unsure, keep reading and once we dig deeper into the formula, you'll know which piece is the right starting point for you.

Warning: Do not make too many changes at once or move on too quickly! Trust me on this one. You have my permission, in fact my orders, to go slowly. Like super silly slow. As in, the one change you start with should feel totally doable and even a little too basic. Perfect! You're in the right spot.

We want to build momentum with easy wins, especially in the beginning.

If you start with the hardest thing first and/or try to add a whole bunch of new things to (or remove things from) your life, you'll get burnt out, overwhelmed, and eventually your motivation won't be enough to keep you going anymore. You'll be done. Instead of all of the changes staying in place, making a positive difference, none of them will last and you'll be back where you started. All-or-nothing usually ends up as nothing sooner or later.

You see, you haven't failed. It's not your fault. It's not lack of willpower. It's the weight loss and diet industry that has failed you. The plans, programs, and diets you've tried have failed. That's why this approach is different. It is based on psychology, behavior change, and my own real life experience (both personal and professional).

The foundation underneath the four part formula is mindset. Your mindset is made up of your mental health, your emotions, and your stress level. Knowing that you are NOT a weak failure is crucial. More on mindset soon, but please be kind and gentle on yourself as you dig into this information and begin applying it to your life.

The key is to keep it simple. If you feel overwhelmed, take a step back and master your current plan before adding on a new step. You don't need to change everything at once—that doesn't work long term. This is not a temporary plan that has a start and end date. This is your plan that you can live with indefinitely, or at least until it's not working anymore and you tweak it again.

Look for the low hanging fruit—the one thing that's easiest to grab and would make the biggest difference. Focus on what matters most right now. Do not rearrange your whole life to make it fit into a plan. Find a plan that fits into your life. Don't get me wrong, you will need to make changes— that's why you're reading this book. You want a change. You need change. You will change— slowly. One baby step at a time. Small, consistent steps forward are better than one giant leap forward followed by a bigger leap backward. Keep it simple. Simple and small. Small steps. Simple steps. Ya feel me? If you're with me and excited about doing this, really doing this once and for all, keep reading. It's about to get good!

To help you with your first small, simple step, I've put together some resources for your fitness journey, which are free for you here: www.fitdamentalsbook.com

FITNESS MYTHS THAT ARE KEEPING YOU STUCK

Let's get right into several popular thoughts in fitness and bust the myths. I want you to know what this book is not about before we get too much further. If you're looking for math equations, percentages, or any other precise, specific formula or plan, then this is not the book for you. If you're looking for a short cut or a way to lose 10 pounds this week, then this is not for you. But if you ARE looking for the truth and simple, basic strategies to help you feel great, then keep reading.

Myth number 1: It's all a matter of calories in versus calories out: eat less/move more.

The common practice to lose weight is to move more (exercise to burn calories) and eat less (go on a diet). In theory this should work, and it often does, at first. There are many problems with this myth. Let's discuss a few of the most common.

First, many dieters (especially women) are already eating a low calorie diet. Eating less is not a good option for these women even if they don't move more. Add in exercise and their bodies freak out (my term, not the technical term for what actually happens). Basically, you're asking your body to do more with less. Our bodies are smarter than we are. They catch on quick and adapt. All your body wants to do is help you survive—at any cost. You may lose weight the first time you try this method. Maybe even the second or third, but eventually it will not work anymore. Your body will have adapted. This is when plateaus and frustration kick in and we look for quick fixes out of desperation.

Another thing that happens with low calorie eating is a lack of nutrients. If you're not eating much, you're not getting the benefits of all the fiber, energy, and nutrients your body needs in order to function at its best. Speaking of energy, how do you expect to have energy for this added movement without enough calories? Calories are not evil. They are not your enemy. They are a unit of energy. They are life. They are vitally important.

Finally, the last point I want to make on the low calorie myth is that not all calories are created equal. I'd rather eat 500 calories worth of healthy nutrients than 300 calories worth of processed, packaged, man-made junk and/or "diet foods." For example, I'd much rather snack on an apple with almond butter (which has carbs, fat, and high calories—gasp!) than some "health food" bar, frozen diet meal, or anything made in a factory. Quality counts. Your body doesn't do math when you eat. It's not counting to be sure you're under your calorie goal for the day. Give it better quality ingredients to work with and it will work better for you. You really ARE what you eat.

Now, as noted, there is a small amount of truth to this myth. There is a reason it works for some, especially the first time. You do need to create a deficit in your energy demands (which basically means burning more than you consume). I know it sounds like I'm contradicting myself, but hear me out. You can create a small deficit through smart nutrition choices and increasing your exercise efforts without starving, feeling deprived, and/ or exercising for hours. It is possible to change your body without a large calorie deficit, but that's beyond the scope of this book. Just trust that you will not be over-exercising and undereating anymore!

Myth 2: You need to be hungry and avoid your favorite foods to lose weight.

As stated in Myth 1, you do NOT need to starve yourself to lose weight. In fact, that can be much more harmful than helpful. Now, you will need to make some changes with your food choices. That's a given. What you are doing or have done in the past isn't working. We will get into more nutrition info soon, so hang in there. Until then, rest assured that you will still be able to enjoy some fun foods once in a while. You will be able to eat enough to satisfy your hunger and have a few treats so you don't feel hungry, deprived, or miserable. We all know the "I'm on a diet" crankiness, and it's not pretty. No more diets!

Myth 3: Insert whatever latest and greatest supplement, shake, diet, detox, or gimmick everyone is talking about.

The myth that you NEED a certain supplement or a specific diet, or my least favorite, a pill that will help you magically lose weight with no effort, is not only wrong, it's harmful. It's hurting your body and it's also hurting your mind. When you fall for these gimmicks and are not successful with them, you think it's your fault. You think that you've failed once again. A loser who can't even lose weight with "the magic fill-in-the-blank." It's not you. It's the multi-billion dollar industry preying on your deepest desires. The method failed—not you. It's not that all diets, plans, supplements, *et cetera*, are bad or harmful, but if it didn't get you where you wanted to go, then it failed you.

Buyer beware! The fitness industry is not regulated. Make sure whatever you try is from a reputable source. Better yet, learn how to improve your health without short term diets or expensive supplements. If it sounds too good to be true, it probably is. If it's making unbelievable claims of huge weight loss in a short time, run away and run away fast! The ability to lose weight fast is another myth all on its own. You cannot burn fat and sculpt a strong, healthy body in a few days or even weeks. It takes time. If you lose a large amount of weight in a short amount of time, it's not fat—at least not a lot of fat. It's probably mostly water and muscle. You do NOT want to lose muscle. There may be well-meaning, honest, solid people out there with claims that actually work, but they are few and far between. Be skeptical. Be a detective and find your own methods. One of my mottos is: If you cannot do it long term, do not even start. Bottom line: Do what you know works for you. Stick to tried and true principles that can be followed indefinitely. (Like eating more veggies.

That never goes out of style) :) Stick around and you'll see how you can make your own plan that will work specifically for you.

Myth 4: You don't have time.

This is more of an excuse than a myth, but I want to bust it right off the bat because it's the number one reason people do not exercise regularly. It does take time. I'm not going to lie and say this will be effortless, but it can be done in less time than you may think. You do not need to spend an hour or more every day in the gym—you don't even need a gym at all. You don't need to cook gourmet meals from scratch. If it's important to you, you'll make the time to do what needs to be done. I'm not making light of this issue. I realize how crazy life can be. I know you're stressed out, tired, and running on empty. Trust the process and know that when you make a few changes, you'll have more energy and you'll be more productive and ready to handle all your other stuff. You can do it, and if I have anything to say about it, you will not sacrifice sleep for it, since burning the candle at both ends doesn't work long term either. The good news is you will not have to get up at stupid o'clock to make it happen! That's the key—you will never *find* the time; you will *make* the time. Scheduling, planning, and committing to your plan is key! Make time. Make it a priority. You may need to let something go, in order to fit it in—girl, that's a whole 'nother conversation—we will talk about your priorities and making yourself one of those priorities soon. Make it happen. You make time for other people's needs all the time. It's time to make time for your own needs. It's not selfish. It's the best thing you can do for your loved ones. They want a happier, healthier you too.

Myth 5: Exercise must be horrible and feel like torture to be effective.

I think you know where I stand on this one. Yes, exercise can be very uncomfortable and some things are unpleasant. However, you do not have to do horrible, torturous workouts to get results. My number one goal when training clients and teaching classes is to make it fun. If it's not enjoyable, you will not come back. That's human nature. If you enjoy it, you'll want to do it again. If you are miserable, you're not going to stick with it. There are so many different workout programs out there, there's no need to do something you don't enjoy. Keep reading to find out the best types for your goals and keep trying new workouts, instructors, and trainers until you find what you like. Side note: If you're too comfortable—as in not challenged, then it probably won't give you great results. You need to find something challenging, effective, and fun. It IS possible. You'll get there soon. I promise.

Myth 6: Cardio (like walking or using an elliptical) is the best for burning fat.

This myth makes me crazy! It's based on some truth and some research done many years ago about heart rate levels and fat burning. However, we've learned a lot since then and while slower paced cardio has its benefits and should be included in a healthy plan, it's not what is going to shape, tone, and change your body. If you're short on time, steady state cardio at a low intensity (like a long walk) is not the best use of it. We'll talk about fitness in a later chapter so you'll know what workouts are more efficient for burning fat, especially when short on time.

Myth 7: You can spot reduce your trouble spots.

We're saving my least favorite myths for last. This myth continues to live on because people create workouts, programs, and plans for specific body parts; i.e. get abs in 30 days, or a plan specific for love handles, or whatever else you may want to target. And because you can build and shape your muscles, which can change the shape of your body, there is a belief that targeting your trouble zones is all you need to do. Fat does not come off one spot alone. It doesn't come off where you want it to. It comes off all over, and it's largely influenced by genetics. If you don't like your stomach and all you do is exercises for your stomach (been there, done that), yes, your stomach muscles will get stronger, but if you need to lose fat, you'll never see those stronger muscles. Once again, hang in there until we get to the fitness chapter, but for now the bottom line is you need an all over program that works your whole body, not just the trouble zones.

Myth 8 (my least favorite): You're unhappy because you're fat and/or when you lose weight, then you'll be happy.

I get it. I've been there. It is easier to accept yourself when your reflection doesn't repulse you. You think you need to lose weight first and then you will like yourself more. I'm going to gently disagree and try to convince you to think differently. You see, when you start making yourself a priority and taking care of yourself, you begin to like yourself more, whether you've lost any weight or not. That doesn't mean you settle for less than you deserve. It doesn't mean you don't aim for bigger, better things and keep making new goals. But it does mean that you're not trying to lose weight only because you hate yourself—you're doing it because you like yourself (dare I say love yourself) and know you deserve better.

YEARS OF BODY HATE

Who am I and why should you listen to me? Great questions. I would be asking the same questions if I were you. It seems too good to be true. Simple tips and a back to basics approach that promises results no matter where you're at or what you've tried before? You have a right to be skeptical. I'd be skeptical too. You've heard lots of promises from fitness companies and health products. There are lots of people in the fitness industry just out to make a profit at your expense. It's a delicate, sensitive subject and unfortunately, there are people out there who are preying on your pain and emotions.

I'm different. I'm not selling anything here. I'm sharing real life experience, struggles, and principles that work. You don't ever have to buy a thing from me for it to work for you (except maybe this book). This is not a fancy sales brochure or commercial. This is not a gimmick to sell you my products, services, or latest and greatest new thing. (You are more than welcome to purchase my services, but they are not necessary for this to work.) I didn't get into fitness to become rich (wrong profession for that). I am here because it's my passion and my purpose. I am here to help you avoid wasting another day on things that don't work. I'm here to help you get to the body of your dreams as simply and quickly as possible. I am here because I care.

Here's why I'm so passionate about helping you learn to live as healthy as possible, as simply as possible: I've been in your shoes—or at least a pair of shoes very similar to yours. I've struggled with my weight since I was a kid. I've been insecure, depressed, and very out of shape. I've tried too many diets to name. I tried many different types of exercise. I was successful in losing weight many times, but I also gained it back many times. That is, until I learned the things I'm going to share with you. I've figured out the biggest, most overlooked pieces. I learned to make it work for my life instead of changing my life to make my diet work. I learned how awesome and precious our bodies are and what they are capable of. I learned to stop hating my body and start appreciating it. You see, when you focus on your faults and weaknesses, that's all you see. When you focus on your strengths, that's what you'll see and that's what you'll get.

But I'm getting ahead of myself. Let's back up to why you should believe me. Have you ever told someone your biggest, deepest, darkest moments? Magnify that and imagine sharing it with the world. Deep breath time. (For me, but you can take one too!) This is hard but I want to let you into my mind and my world. You should know I am an extremely introverted person and I've never shared these stories—like, with anyone. So why am I telling you? Because we are more alike than you know. I am fit now. I am a trainer, instructor, coach, and overall healthy person now. Looking at me you might not think I can relate to you (even though I have the stretch marks, loose skin, cellulite, and scars to prove it). I can relate, and I do. More than you know.

I've been so overwhelmed with trying to find something to wear that the thought of opening my closet has sent me back to bed. I've cancelled plans because I was too fat and disgusted with myself to be seen in public. I've held back affection and love to my hubby because I didn't want my body to be seen or touched. I literally failed gym class in high school and had to go to summer school because I was too self-conscious and embarrassed to participate in front of my classmates. Yup, I'm the girl who sat on the sidelines and chose to fail Phys. Ed.

Does any of that sound familiar? I thought so. We may have different stories but the experiences and the feelings are similar. If you struggle with your weight (you wouldn't be reading this book if you didn't), we are connected. We have fought the same fights and we are in the same battle together. It doesn't matter if you have 10 pounds or 100 pounds to lose. The emotions are similar no matter where you are starting from. I've worked with women of different ages, backgrounds, and sizes, and we all have the same things in common: when we don't feel good about our bodies, and we are not taking care of ourselves, everything suffers. We put others first until we don't even recognize ourselves anymore.

It's time to take care of you! It's time to put your oxygen mask on before you can assist anyone else. It's time to fill your cup with love and self-care so you have love to give to the important people in your life. It's time to have more energy, more patience, more joy!

It is possible. It may be hard to believe. Maybe you've tried so many times, you're doubtful it can ever work. Maybe this is the last straw and you're ready to give up. Wherever you're at and however you're feeling today, hang in there. Please don't ever give up on yourself. I want the best for you. By the end of this book, you will want the best for yourself too.

Back to those stories I promised to share with you. I've put off sharing them for long enough. The first story I want to share with you is not something I take lightly. Please know that I understand psychological disorders, and I know how serious eating disorders are. I am sharing this so you will know just how low and desperate I was.

When I was in middle school, probably about age 12 or 13, I desperately wanted to be bulimic. Seriously. I know how disturbing that sounds, but it's true. I tried everything to make myself vomit many, many times, but I couldn't do it. One more thing I was a failure at—at least that's how it felt at the time. It seemed like such a simple solution. I could still binge on junk and then "get rid of it" like it had never happened. I thought it was the best of both worlds: eat junk and be "skinny." Little did I know then how serious and life threatening it was.

I still thank God to this day that I failed at bulimia. I'll never forget the feeling of pushing my toothbrush down my throat, praying to be able to vomit the massive amount of junk in my stomach (most likely a combination of Doritos, Pepsi, Devil Dogs, and Blow Pops—I was addicted to Blow Pops). I can still feel the cold porcelain and see the clean, empty toilet water, feeling disappointed once again. I couldn't do it. Failure again. I cried over that ivory toilet many times.

So, vomiting wasn't the answer, but I couldn't stop my binges and love of sweets of all kinds. I used to joke that I didn't just inherit my Nana's sweet tooth, I inherited an entire mouthful of sweet teeth. Oh, you should have seen the treats we enjoyed together. (Candy corn anyone?)

So, maybe not eating was the answer. Maybe, just maybe I could go without eating for long periods and only eat occasionally. I would save my favorite things for when I allowed myself to eat. That didn't work well either. Not eating was harder than forcing myself to vomit. Especially when all of my favorite junk foods were easily available right in the kitchen. (I inherited my dad's appetite, but not his fast metabolism.) And we all know once you start eating Doritos, you don't stop at one serving. You stop when half the bag is gone. (Or, the whole bag, who are we kidding!) Then wash it down with soda.

OK, I wasn't successful in controlling my eating to lose weight, so maybe I could out-exercise my food intake. You know, like if I ate a bunch of junk, I could just exercise until those calories were gone. I tried. We will talk more about calories and diet/exercise soon. For now, just know that it's not that simple. You can't really undo one with the other. I promised you simple solutions, and they are coming, but working out to burn more calories while undereating and consuming too few calories is NOT one of them.

I remember wanting desperately to be Denise Austin or one of the background ladies behind Gilad in *Bodies in Motion*. I would come home after school and find workout programs on TV. I wanted to look like them, move like them, do what they could do, and really, just be athletic. I liked how it felt when I could do something physical (like swim, roller skate, ride my bike, or make it through a TV workout). I just never wanted to do it in public where people could see me and make fun of my fat body. It seems so funny to me now that I am a trainer and teach fitness classes. (Like in public, in the FRONT of the room where everyone can see me! It's nuts!) I always felt judged, bullied, and insecure. I pretended I didn't want to play, just to avoid being made fun of.

While I'm still not Denise Austin, I've found my own way of being fit and enjoying exercise. (Even in public!) You can too, even if you never go public with it. I spent many years, even recently, working out alone at home. A gym is not required to get fit. Let me say that again:

A gym is not required to get fit.

You can do it in the comfort and privacy of your own home. (Although, I still think working out on the beach, like Gilad and Denise have done in their careers, is the way to go. That really does make it so much more appealing. :) Maybe we will work out on the beach together someday.)

My time with Denise and Gilad on TV after school may have prevented me from being extremely obese, but it didn't prevent me from being overweight and insecure. In fact, as I got older, my body image got worse. I became depressed in high school. Long story short, not only did I fail that gym class (and have to spend four weeks in summer school on the track to make it up), but I even ended up dropping out of high school. There are a number of factors I won't go into, but the bottom line is I was depressed and extremely low on self-esteem. I had been teased, called names, and picked on for being the fat kid. It hurts. I get it. I know the pain you feel. Intimately. I know.

The good news is your past doesn't define you. It's only part of the story. You have control over the rest of the story. Your family history and genetics do not define you. What others think or say about you certainly does NOT define you. You are in charge, my friend and that's a good thing. A very good thing. It's liberating to know that you are in the driver's seat. You can live the life of your dreams. You can take control and do amazing things with your body and your life. It's not too late, you're not too fat, and you're definitely not too lazy, out of shape, or whatever else you may think! I ended up going back to school to earn a degree (summa cum laude, thank you very much!) and I have several fitness certifications. You really can do anything you put your mind to.

I'll avoid the super cheesy, "If I can do it, you can do it!" spiel. What I really want you to know is that *anything is possible*. I've seen it. Not just in my life, but in the lives of my clients, friends, and peers. The sky's the limit and no one can stop you when you want it and believe it. You are worth it. You deserve it. You can do it, and you WILL do it! Ready? Let's go!

MINDSET

Before we get into specifics, let's talk about what matters more than diet, exercise, or anything else. This is the stuff that will make or break you. If you've tried to lose weight before and either were not successful in losing it, or perhaps you lost the weight but then gained some or all of it back, this may be the critical piece you were missing. And it's not your fault. Most weight loss plans focus on the actions, like exercise and meal plans, without making sure you're ready and able to follow through on the plans. The very best plan in the world will not work if you're not ready, or able, to follow it. Sure, we all know how to lose weight—it's not rocket science. We've done it before—more than once. The critical piece is learning to change your mindset about diet and weight loss. When you have the right mindset, you'll bounce back from setbacks faster (we all have setbacks), and you'll stop yo-yoing up and down. You'll be in the fight for good. You'll be prepared and ready to make changes and keep moving forward.

Gratitude

The first tip in creating a positive mindset is Gratitude. Many experts recommend writing in a Gratitude journal daily, listing things you are thankful for. I personally find daily entries a little overwhelming and it takes the joy out of it for me. It becomes just another thing on my list of things to do each day. Instead, I spend time each morning in prayer, which is another form of gratitude. Experiment and find what works for you.

Whatever method you choose, the point is to focus on the things in your life you are grateful for. This may seem basic and silly at first. You'll inevitably write about your family, friends, and other loved ones in the beginning, but then it gets harder. In order not to keep repeating yourself, you have to dig deep and get creative. I've been known to be grateful for coffee, my favorite yoga mat, the sunroof in my car, PiYo, and avocados (among other, deeper things I assure you, but we can be thankful for coffee and avocados too). Spend some time on this daily, or at least weekly. It's been shown in research to be very helpful in improving happiness. It is not possible to be grateful and anxious at the same time. My intention for you is to take your mind off of what you do not have, and place it on all the good things in your life. You may surprise yourself how many good things you have once you start focusing on them.

Along the same lines as being grateful, your next tip is to focus on what you *can* do instead of what you cannot do. So often I hear women put themselves down about what they can't do (or think they can't do). For example, instead of, "I have no upper body strength, I'll never be able to do a full push up," switch it up to something like, "I've never had much upper body strength, but I'm getting stronger. My half push ups are getting better. Soon I'll be able to attempt a full one."

If you have an injury or limitation, don't spend your time and energy thinking about it. Think about all the things you can still do. We see this with amputees who continue to be active and accomplish amazing physical feats, in spite of their handicaps. There really are no excuses—only challenges.

So, my friend, the next time you catch yourself complaining about something you cannot do or something you do not have, stop immediately.

Think about all of your blessings. Focus on the positive. No matter how badly you feel, there is always something to be thankful for. You have life, breath, and another day to take a step toward your dreams.

Fitness is, first, an internal decision

Health, fitness, and weight loss start from the inside. Once you start taking care of yourself, you'll start to feel better. When you start to feel better, you'll want to keep taking care of yourself. It's a positive circular pattern that builds in momentum. Once you build that momentum and start feeling great, you won't want to stop, and then the results will come. It starts on the inside.

Once you decide you want more for your life, and you are willing to make yourself a priority, then you won't be fooled by the latest and greatest fads anymore. You won't look for the fastest, easiest way to lose weight—like now! You'll know it's about more than how you look. It's about how you feel. It's about your health. It's your LIFE! It all begins in your mind with your thoughts. Thoughts lead to emotions. Emotions lead to actions. Actions bring results (good or bad). If you're focused on the actions without addressing the thoughts and emotions, then it's only logical that it won't work.

The actions aren't the problem. You know what to do. We all know how to lose weight. The *how* isn't the problem. It's the *why* that's the bigger issue.

Your *why* will keep you going on the tough days. Your *why* will push you when the scale doesn't cooperate and you want to give up. Your *why* is everything. It's the internal motivation to keep going. You don't need to search for external motivation. You have it within you. Once you have a deep, meaningful, powerful reason to make changes, you'll be able to challenge yourself and make difficult choices (like salad instead of a pizza). Knowing your *why* makes these choices become less of a struggle. You'll no longer need to rely on willpower. You will WANT to make healthy choices. (It's crazy, but it's true.)

Here's an example: Let's say you are going to do this because you're tired of not liking what you see in the mirror. I ask you, why? Because you don't like the way it makes you feel. Why? Because you don't like yourself and it feels bad. Why? Because you take care of everyone else and you've let yourself go so far you don't even recognize yourself anymore. Why? Because you stopped taking care of yourself. Why? Because you don't feel worthy of the effort. Why? You get the idea.... Keep going until you cry. Seriously.

Weight loss and body image issues are not about diet and exercise. Not really. Those are important pieces in dealing with it, but the underlying factor isn't that you don't know what exercises to do or what to eat. It's more complex than that. It's about being internally motivated. You can seek out inspiration to help fill your mind with positive thoughts, but ultimately, motivation comes from within. Inspiration can give you a spark, but you have all the power you need already. You just need to learn to harvest it. Put another way, inspiration is external (outside sources) and motivation is internal. You need a healthy dose of both. I'm not knocking outside inspiration by any means. (Although, be careful whom you follow for inspiration. Sometimes it can backfire if it's too extreme.) However, even the most inspirational post, picture, video, quote, whatever, won't last long if you don't find your own internal spark.

Let's dig into your *why*. It's time to find your own powerhouse already inside you. You are your own pusher, coach, and get-er-done-er. If you're distracted by other things right now, deal with them and come back when you can focus. This is serious and it may take some time and a bit of deep thought. Don't be discouraged. You can totally do this. Just please give it your full attention. This really is a huge step towards your goals. It starts now. Ready? Let's jump in!

We are going to find your *why*. Your reason for wanting to do this. Your motivation for making tough choices and challenging yourself. Why? But really, why? No, I mean really, really *why*? Try not to use too many external reasons, like looking a certain way (i.e. I want to see my abs). That is just not deep enough to keep you going on the hard days. We all have hard days. They're inevitable. How will you handle them? Will you give up or will you keep going? You will keep going because you'll have internal motivation and a deep, meaningful reason.

Is it for your kids? Maybe your doctor is making you lose weight? Maybe you're just tired of being tired. That's a great start. Think about those reasons for a moment.

Stop and think.

Why did you pick up this book? Why do you want to do this? Why are you going to work out when you don't feel like it? Why? Why? WHY? Did you come up with something that made you emotional? If not, keep asking why. Be like an annoying two-year-old toddler and keep asking why, why, why? Keep drilling down until you hit a tender spot. You need to feel it in your heart—not your head. If the thought of living long enough to see your grandkids have kids causes you to tear up, you're on the right track. If one of your parents died of a preventable disease and your *why* is to live longer and end the cycle, you're on the right track. We're digging deep for tenderness here.

The extra weight is a symptom of something bigger. Something deeper. You see the consequences on the surface (and in the mirror), but the real issues are underneath, in a safe place you've kept hidden from others, and from yourself, for too long. This may take some time. Really sit with this for a while. If you don't get down to the deep stuff, this will all be just another short-term plan you follow for a while, lose a little weight and then gain it back. I just can't tolerate that and neither should you. You are worth more!

You are worth the time and effort to figure this out. If you find yourself getting too upset or having depressive thoughts, please talk to a counselor or someone trained to help you sort through it. Weight loss is an emotional journey and it will reveal things about yourself you maybe didn't want to discover. But self-discovery needs to happen if you want lasting results and complete freedom from your weight and self-esteem struggles. Food habits and body image can be difficult things to address. You need to be honest with yourself and open to changing your thoughts and attitude.

It will take effort and work. It will take time. But it will be worth it. You are worth it. Your family is worth it. They deserve the best version of you possible, and so do you. I beg you not to skip this! I know you want to get into the details of what, when, and how to lose weight, but I promise you this is the foundation. Bypassing this will not work for long. You may have temporary success—the formula does work, whether you do this part or not—but it won't last.

We are like toddlers who need discipline. Not because we are bad and need punishment, but because we want what is best for ourselves. Discipline, when done with love, shows care, concern, and respect. Taking care of ourselves is difficult. It takes time, effort, and commitment.
We want instant gratification and quick fixes or we get cranky. Just like the toddler, we need boundaries. This is tough. You may want to give up, throw yourself on the floor, pound your fists, and say screw it. Please, don't! If you want to learn, if you want to grow into a healthier version of yourself, you must resist the urge to give into the tantrum and stay in it for the long run. You are now focused on long term benefits, not short term desires.

Your motivation comes from the desire to stop playing this game. Get off the rollercoaster and come on a journey to a better life. You will still have ups and downs—that's part of life —but the extremes will be gone. No more starting over or "dieting." (That's a bad word in my vocabulary.) You can do this and it's simpler than you imagine. Not easy, but simple.

Your health is a priority. It is priceless and deserves both time and effort. I'd like it to be near the top of your list of priorities, as in unless there is an emergency or unforeseen event, your daily healthy habits will happen. You will never be any younger than you are today—don't waste another day feeling less than you're capable of. Schedule time for it. Have a plan, find someone to hold you accountable, and do not blow it off! You deserve to show up for you! You are worth the time and the effort.

Let's get straight to the truth. No more wasting time. No more games. No more foolish gimmicks, tricks, or desperate measures. NO MORE hating our bodies. It's like marriage and parenting. It's hard. Really hard. But so worth it. The good far outweighs the bad. It takes effort, commitment, and love—lots of love.

Finally, if all else fails to motivate you, my number one reason for caring for my body is not about me at all. It's a symbol of my faith. Our bodies are created and they are amazing. We are called to take care of them and treat them well. We are called to use them in serving others and the world. We cannot do that if we are tired, weak, and sick. That, my friend, is your ultimate source of motivation, inspiration, and power. Remember that you have access to the King of the Universe anytime you need Him, and He cares for you. Live the life you were born to live—serve with passion, purpose, and energy. When you are weak, He is strong.

Setting the right types of goals

The foundation for developing motivation and staying in the game long term is to establish your internal drive from the start. Intrinsic, or internal, motivation works better and lasts longer than any external motivation. That's good news! Basically, you can motivate yourself. Now that you know your *why*, let's talk about how to put it into practice with some goals!

By switching your focus to intrinsic (internal) goals rather than extrinsic (external) goals, you are able to keep going when the scale, or the mirror, doesn't cooperate. Your motivation is bigger than outward appearance. Your health (indeed, your life) is more valuable than how you look. Whenever you find yourself slipping into old habits (they die hard), remember your *why* and your intrinsic desires for a healthy, happy life.

Knowing your why and having meaningful goals is the foundation this formula is built on. It's vital to making sure you don't give up. I'm making this stuff as simple as possible, but let's be honest:

It's not easy.

It's easy to eat whatever you want in the moment and lie around all day. It's hard to eat well and work out. It's HARD. It takes commitment, sacrifice, and love. Lots of love. We discipline our kids because we love them. We want what is best for them. We need to discipline ourselves too. Not because we are bad and need punishment but because we want what is best for ourselves. Discipline, when done with love, shows care, concern, and respect.

You deserve love, care, and respect. You are worth the effort. Take the time to build this foundation before jumping into the details.

Since we're on the subject of goals, let's dig into that a little further. I tend to be a goal-oriented person. I like goals. I set them; I go after them; I reach them (not always); and I set new, bigger ones. I like the thrill of the chase and the sense of accomplishment. If you don't plan out where you want to go and how to get there, how will you know when to celebrate? How will you know if you were successful? How will you know what's working and when it's time to make a change? I believe in goals, like, a lot. But there are ways to set and achieve goals that are empowering and positive, and there are ways that set you up for failure. Let's do it the right way and improve our chance of success significantly.

When setting goals, it's important to remember to make SMART goals. SMART is an acronym that stands for Specific, Measurable, Attainable; Realistic (this one is up for debate—some use Relevant); and Time-bound. Let's break each piece of that down so you'll know if your goals are SMART or not.

Specific. Specific means exactly that. Specificity. Details. No vague fuzziness. Your brain needs details—very specific details. Goals with words such as "more," "better," or "less" won't cut it. Do not set a goal to eat better. What does better mean? What will that look like on a daily/weekly basis? If your goal is to lose weight, get specific with what that really means. This usually involves numbers. I will lose 10 pounds—that's specific. I will eat at least 3 servings of veggies every day— that's specific. I will eat less junk food—that's not specific (I was testing to see if you were paying attention).

Now that you know you need specifics in order to have solid goals, let's talk about the M: Measurable. Again, just like specific, the measurable part involves details—usually numbers. Instead of I want to lose weight, change it to I want to lose ___ pounds. There is a saying that states 'you can't manage what you don't measure.' In order to know if you've hit your goal or not, you need a way to measure results. Whether it's a goal for workouts each week, veggies each day, hours of sleep each night, or any other goals you may decide to set for yourself, make sure you have some way of measuring results. (Hint: Try measuring with something other than a scale.) :)

The next step in your SMART goal is to make sure it is A: Attainable. Sure, you can set a very specific, measurable goal to run a 10K, but if you've never run a mile, that might be not an attainable goal for you (at least not yet). I want you to dream really, really, big, but keep a moderate amount of reality in your goals to avoid disappointment and failure. Are you trying to reach an unattainable, unrealistic version of yourself because it looks good on someone else, or because you used to look a certain way? The best bet is to set goals you're fairly certain you can reach—at least for now. (Bigger, scarier, and less realistic goals can come later!) You want to set yourself up for a win. Heck yeah, you can work out for 20 minutes 4 days a week—no brainer. You just need to make sure it's a goal moving you forward. Don't make it so attainable that it's not a stretch. Make sure you're challenging yourself just enough to make progress without getting overwhelmed.

Which brings us to Realistic (or Relevant). This one is a slight spin off of Attainable. You may decide that losing 30 pounds is attainable, as in you do actually have 30 pounds to lose. However, it may not be realistic at this moment. Maybe you're going through a really stressful time, or you have some underlying health issues, or many other reasons why 30 pounds, at least right now, is not realistic. Start smaller. Start with 10. If you'd like to use Relevant instead, decide if that goal is really relevant to you right now. Maybe your goal involves wearing a certain outfit (bikini, anyone?), but is that really relevant? Do you actually have the item and plans to wear it, or are you dreaming of a someday scenario? I'm not going to encourage you to be realistic very often (dream BIG), but when setting goals, I want you to be set up for success, which involves a good dose of reality. (Boo!)

Finally, you need deadlines. Your goal needs to be Time-bound. When will it happen? How long will it take? When is the cut-off date? You need a time period to make sure you stay on track. When will you assess your Measurement to know if you're successful or not? 30 days? 90 days? Remember to keep your time frame in line with the rest of the details—especially Realistic and Attainable. We all work better under pressure, and we need deadlines to make sure we follow through. Otherwise, you'll keep procrastinating and putting it off until tomorrow, or Monday. Always Monday.

Now that your goals are all SMART and stuff, let's figure out exactly *how* you're going to reach them. See, while it's uber important to know where you want to go, it's even more important to know how you're going to get there. You're not wasting any more time chasing unrealistic goals, and you're not wasting any more time spinning your wheels in the wrong direction. It's time to take this party on the road and move onward and upward my friend.

My biggest, most favorite tip when it comes to goal setting, is to focus on action rather than results. But wait, didn't we just go through a whole section on setting goals with SMART results? Yes, yes we did. And it's important. Don't skip that part. For real, go back and create your SMART goal(s).

Focus on the action steps

Once you know where you want to go (i.e. once you have your SMART goal), let's peel it back and figure out how you will get there. By shifting your attention to the actions needed to get there, rather than the destination, you'll be able to break things down into smaller, simple, easy win steps. Once you do that, you can look at those individual steps as small, measurable goals that you can track, so you'll know if you're doing what you said you would do or not.

So, my friend, what are your action steps? What can you do to get where you want to go? What activities, habits, or behaviors will get you to your ultimate goal? As noted, now's the time to stop focusing on the destination and start focusing on the journey. (Cheesy, I know, but it works.) What will your journey look like? There are so many possibilities, or paths to take, to get to your goal. Start with one action, and keep adding new ones as you adapt, learn, and get closer to your dreams. Action baby—take action!

I'm going to drive this one home a little more. Bear with me. It's really important that you get this. Not just in your head, but in your heart. I need you to believe me on this one because the result is fabulous. You know where you want to go and that's huge. You've even been SMART about it and set some pretty awesome goals that you are confident you can reach. Now, stop thinking about them. Stop. I know it goes against everything you've ever been taught about reaching your goals. But if you really want to be successful this time, trust me on this. Don't think about the 10 pounds, or the fill-in-the-blank goal you set for yourself. Think about actions you will do each and every day. The goal is still there. You're not abandoning it. It's just waiting for you on the other side of action. Take action, every day, every meal, every bite. Action will get you to your desired destination—thinking, dreaming, and wishing will not.

You may be sensing a theme here—focus on what you are doing and take small, consistent steps each day. Baby steps. Steps are *action.* Even small, baby steps will move you forward. If you've ever trained for a long distance walk or run, you know it's more about the preparation, training, and small, daily things you did to prepare than the actual event. Your finish line (goal) is the same way. It's the small, daily training (actions) you do each day that will get you to your finish line. Consistency and small, actionable steps are key.

So, now go back and reevaluate your goals and your action steps. Are they still SMART? Do you have action steps (things you will do to get where you want to go)? Are the actions small enough? Are they bite-sized, baby steps that are totally doable? Are they maintainable, long term? If so, you're on the right track. If not, spend some time really thinking about what you want, why you want it, and how you will get there. If you still don't know what actions to take, start with the basics: drink water, move your body at least 3 days a week, eat at least 3 veggies a day, etc. Once you have at least a few solid action items, it's time for the next step. Check out the Action plan and Appendix at the back of this book for help to get started.

Now that you have action steps, you need a plan. It's great to know what to do, but now you need to actually DO it. This is when your organizational skills come in handy. Create a schedule for your workouts, and anything else you need help tracking. Literally put it on your calendar. Start with one week (or one day) at a time. What will you do (training session, group class, on demand work out, walk at the park)? When will you do it? Put it in writing. Schedule it like a real appointment with an important person (because it is). Now, if you value being spontaneous, free, and unscheduled, I get it. I do too, but some things require planning and commitment. Your health, especially your workouts, is one of those things. Let's face it, it won't just happen, no matter how determined you are, without a plan.

You may need very specific, detailed plans listing out every exercise and every set and every meal with every ingredient (that's too much for me, but it might work for you), or you may just need to write general overviews such as: full body workout with Jenn, or chili for dinner. Simple. To the point. Write it out in advance and follow through. Once you have action steps and a plan, it's time to go Nike style and "Just Do It"!

Now, this is where it gets hard. Everyone spends so much time and money trying to figure out how to do this stuff and they neglect the hardest part— actually doing it. This is where my second favorite tip comes into play: accountability. It's time to tell someone and get some outside support. Recruit people who will hold you up and encourage you.

Accountability is one of the main reasons personal training works so well for some people. It's not really about the workout (shhh, keep that secret between us). It's the appointment, the money you spent, and the fact that someone is expecting you to show up and do the work, someone other than yourself, or your BFF who lets you off the hook every time you cancel.

However, you don't need to hire a personal trainer to tap into the power of the accountability factor. You may even be able to use your BFF as an accountability buddy, if she will actually make you follow through and show up. Some accountability partners turn into excuse validating complaint partners (don't let this happen to you), while others motivate and challenge each other (this is what you want in a good buddy).

Posting on social media or making an announcement to your family can be a good way to hold yourself accountable. Making your goals and your action steps public can be very motivating. If you've announced that you're giving up sugar and are joining a gym, you're much less likely to dive face first into the sweet treats at the office (or function, or, you know, like, Tuesday).

Which brings up the topic of social media. This one is loaded, but let me just briefly say, be careful. Be careful what you share, who you share it with, and who you follow on social media.

Negative people like causing a commotion when they see someone doing something positive. You will attract Debbie Downers. You might even live with them. But there are a lot of very positive, encouraging people in this world. You are not alone and you do not have to listen to the doubters. Surround yourself with positive people who believe in you and push you to be better. Unfollow all negativity. You don't have to let it into your life. Remember that your happiness begins with your thoughts, so choose what you allow into your mind very carefully.

Non-Scale Victories

Finally, my last tip for reaching your goals is to celebrate every step of the way. I call this Non-Scale Victories (NSV). I didn't make it up—it's a thing. Just as you focus on your action steps to reach your SMART goals, and the actions themselves become tiny, measurable goals (for example, I ate 5 veggies today—I hit my goal!), now the changes in your health become the wins. Pay attention to how well you sleep, if your skin clears up, if your joints are less achy, if you can push harder in your workout, etc. Look for small wins and claim them as victories! Don't wait until you reach the finish line to be proud of yourself. Be proud of every mile marker along the way.

As we wind down this section on goals, if you're still unsure where to start and what actions to take, ask yourself: What is biggest thing in my way now? What is holding me back? What one thing could I do (or not do) to get moving forward? Make one change to improve that thing. Stick with it until it's working, and then add the next thing. Start with the basics first (water, veggies, activity) before focusing on smaller details (specific nutrition strategies like low carb, specific training plans, etc.).

Remember to keep it simple! Do something. Do anything. Any improvement is better than nothing. Any step forward will help you reach your goals. You don't need to change everything at once—that doesn't work long term. This is not a temporary plan that has a start and end date. This is your plan that you can live with indefinitely, until it's not working anymore and you need to tweak it again. Nothing is set in stone forever and always. It's a living, working, changing "plan" for lack of a better term. It's your life. It's your health. We are trying to lower your stress and improve your well-being, not add more stress with hard to follow rules. If you ever feel overwhelmed, stressed out, or confused by this program, then take a step back and focus on just one thing at a time and stay with it until it's working before you change anything else. You'll know it's working when you look forward to it instead of dreading it. For example, no one needs to remind me to drink lots of water anymore. I crave it and feel cranky without it. I don't drink because I *have* to, I drink it because I *want* to.

WATER

This first step in your new life of healthy habits begins with drinking more water. If you were paying attention in the goal setting section, you know that 'more' is not a specific, measurable goal. Therefore, you will need to decide what number to use to track your 'more.' Most people are not hydrated enough and many are slightly dehydrated without even knowing it.

You need more water than you think you do

You have probably heard the advice to drink 64 ounces a day (8 glasses, 8 ounces each). That is not ideal for most people. Don't panic, but I aim for 100-120 ounces (5-6 large water bottles or 12-15 cups) a day. You don't have to start there! You get to choose what your version of 'more water' will look like for you.

Let's start with some newer, more accurate guidelines you can use to determine your water goal. (Oooh, let's make that a thing: #watergoals.) The recommendation, at the moment, is to drink approximately half of your body weight in ounces of water at a minimum. For example, if you weigh 180 pounds, you would aim for at least 90 ounces or 11 to12 cups (because, math: half of 180 is 90). I know we don't want to do math if we don't have to, but this one is simple and once you have your number (#watergoals) you don't have to do it again.

Keep in mind that your number is the minimum recommendation. If you are very active (or it's a hot, humid day) and you sweat a lot, you need more water to offset the perspiration. If you drink anything that dehydrates you (I'm looking at you, coffee), you need to offset the caffeinated drink with an extra serving of water. So, you can see why most people are not getting enough. 64 ounces would be ideal if you weighed 120-130 pounds, don't sweat and don't drink (or eat) anything with caffeine.

The simple test to see if you're drinking enough water

Another simple tip to be sure you're getting enough water is to drink enough so that you NEED to get up and go to the bathroom at least once every couple of hours. The extra benefit to that (besides staying hydrated) is you'll get up and take a short walk to the bathroom, which adds extra steps and activity to your day. Yay, win-win!

While you're in there taking your bathroom breaks, take a peek at the bowl when you're done (TMI, I know, but it's important). You want your urine to be pale yellow. Not so light that it's clear, but not so dark that it's bright or deep in color. The only time it should be dark is just after taking a vitamin or supplement, when you will flush out (literally) the extra nutrients your body doesn't absorb. (Or if you've recently eaten a lot of beets. Yay vegetables!)

The pee test is a very simple way to know if you're drinking enough without having to count, track or measure anything—because you know I'm not about to make you do math! :)

Why is water so important anyway? Why can't you just drink whatever you want? Isn't liquid good enough no matter what type of liquid? Nice try, but no. No, it's not. Water is what your body needs and wants. It might not be what your taste buds want, but it is what you need to feel your best. Every cell in your body needs water to function well. Like everything! You will think more clearly, have healthier hair, skin, and nails, and flush out toxins and other stuff your body needs to get rid of, including fat! It's your sewer system and it needs to keep things moving along. Stagnation is not good.

A simple tip to get more water is to start the day with it. Drink at least one large glass, first thing in the morning before you put anything else in your body. Add a splash of lemon juice or apple cider vinegar for extra detox, and weight loss, benefits. Another tip is to keep a large water bottle with you all day long, so it's right there when you need it (every hour). You can add a splash of flavor to it if you really don't like the flavor of it plain, but humor me and try it—you just might develop a taste for it. Some suggestions for flavoring are to add some fresh fruit, herbs, or spices. Cucumber, mint, citrus, and berries are some of my faves. You can add some seltzer water too if you like the fizz factor. Just be aware that fizz can cause bloating and other problems, so use it as a treat and not your main source of water.

I think you know this already, but just in case it's not clear, make sure you are drinking *water*. Real water. As in H2O. You can flavor it yourself. Do not drink sweetened, artificially flavored, colored, "healthy" water. Once again, if it was made in a factory, it's probably not a high quality, healthy choice, no matter how appealing and healthy the commercials make it seem. If God made it and it's in its natural state (as natural as possible), then you're on the right track.

Drink up my friend and see what a huge difference this one habit can make in how you feel, look, and live. Gulp, gulp!

FOOD

L et's cut right to the bottom line. Healthy food does not come out of factories, packages, boxes, and bags. Real healthy food doesn't make health claims. It doesn't have to. No one has to convince you that spinach, or an apple, is healthy. They don't wrap it up with a bunch of catchy words to show off the health benefits. It's not necessary. You know produce is healthy. That's the bottom line. Eat real food. REAL. FOOD. As in food that grows from the earth—not science experiments that come out of "food" factories. There are some healthy foods made in factories, After all, most of us are not growing and making our own food from scratch. We live in the real world and need to get our food from somewhere. If it's something you could make at home if you had the time and the desire, and it doesn't have extra stuff added to it, then it may be a healthy option.

Now that you know the bottom line, let me back up to explain how this can work for you, and explore a few common, but not well understood, healthy food tips.

Clean Eating has become a popular term recently. It has many different interpretations depending on whom you ask. (The term came from Tosca Reno. Look her up. She's written several books about clean eating.)

Basically, Clean Eating is eating food in as natural a state as possible. No long ingredient lists. No prepared foods or fast food. Whole, real, fresh, nutritious food. There are some finer details to the Clean Eating method, such as pairing protein with carbs and never eating any type of carb by itself, including fruit. I don't get that technical with it. We're keeping it simple, remember? In my mind, an apple by itself, even without protein, is better than chips, candy, or any other snack you may usually reach for.

As noted, one of the standard rules of Clean Eating is to avoid foods with long ingredient lists. Ideally, you'll eat foods without labels and ingredient lists, but it's not realistic to never eat a prepared food item again. When you are eating a premade food, look at the ingredients and aim for 5 items or less, and make sure these items are things you can identify. If you don't know what it is, chances are your body doesn't know what to do with it.

Read the ingredients label

When looking at food packaging, skip the front. The buzz words that catch your eye on the front of the package are not important. The very FIRST thing to look for when examining a food item is the ingredient list. Yup, ingredients FIRST. Not calories, carbs, sodium, or any of the nutrition facts.

When reading the ingredients, look for simple, short lists containing real food. An example would be hummus. It may have 4-6 ingredients, but you know what they are (chickpeas, oil, tahini, etc.) Anything with added sugar, artificial sweeteners or colors is out. Right off the bat. Put it down and walk away!

Quality counts

The nutritional quality of what you put into your body counts more than calories. Quality, quality, quality. Eat highly nutritious foods as much as possible and I guarantee you will feel better. You deserve high octane, top of the line fuel in the amazingly complicated machine you live in. Treat it well. Maintain it better than anything else you own. It has to last a very long time.

We tend to overeat low nutritional quality foods. (Bag full of chips, anyone?) When was the last time you overate broccoli? It just doesn't happen. Low quality foods don't satisfy. They leave us overfed but malnourished. Your body is begging for food high in fiber, vitamins, and minerals.

That brings me to the next tip: Fill up on high fiber, nutrient dense foods as much as possible. This approach is more about adding good, high quality foods into your diet, and less about restricting or eliminating bad, or low quality, foods from your life. When you focus on the good, the lesser options automatically become fewer and farther between. You'll learn to enjoy the taste of fresh, real food and your cravings for junk will diminish without you feeling deprived or restricted. It might sound too good to be true, but I promise it's possible.

The 80/20 rule

You don't have to actually count and track exact percentages, but it's a good rule of thumb to plan for at least 80% of the food you eat to be healthy, clean, quality food, and 20% for indulgences, treats, and special occasions. (Tortilla chips on date night is one of my 20% items.) Keeping your fave "vices" is an important part of creating a healthy lifestyle plan you can stick with long term. A life without things you love is not enjoyable. But a life full of too many treats is not healthy. The magic is in finding the balance between mostly healthy and a few occasional treats just for fun, just because you enjoy them and they make you happy. That's why I love the 80/20 rule. It works for business, it works for most things in life, and it really works when finding your unique Fit Food plan.

If you are an all-or-nothing person, the moderation of 80/20 may not work for you. If you feel you need more discipline to stick to your goals (especially if you're at a plateau) aim for a 90/10 split. 100% doesn't work for long. You need at least a 10% window of "fun foods" to make sure you avoid the Diet Mentality and feelings of deprivation, restriction, and aggravation. I follow something close to 80/20 now (it's an estimate— no calculations needed while eating), but I used to follow a 90/10 rule.

The 90/10 approach worked really well for me, and still does when I feel the need to dial it back in, because when you plan for only 10% fun food and you go overboard and have extra treats, it still ends up around 80/20. If you plan for 80/20, and go overboard, it ends up being 70/30-ish or something like that, at least for me. I'm not good with moderation, so allowing 20% treats can snowball quickly into way too many treats. But allowing 10% is just enough to make me feel like I'm not deprived—I can still eat my fave foods— just not in large quantities. It's small enough to remind me to choose wisely and save it for what I really love.

This is where you experiment and find out your balance point. Just how many indulgences do you really NEED to feel satisfied and how sparingly can you spread them out? You need to choose wisely. Treats add up quickly. Know your off-limit foods—food you just do not trust yourself to eat in moderation. Know what you can savor and walk away from when you need to. Save your fun foods for things you really enjoy. Don't waste it on just anything. Be wise. Be intentional. Plan for it and then enjoy it, really enjoy it, without guilt. No more Diet Mentality!

No calorie-counting

It may go without saying at this point, but if it's not clear already, let me clarify one very important thing: you do NOT need to do math while eating! No calorie counting, no percentages, no complicated spreadsheets that take longer to fill out than it took you to eat the meal! If you are a numbers person, and you really have no idea if you're anywhere close to a healthy diet plan, then tracking for a few days is a good idea. It can be helpful to know where you're at and what needs to change. However, it is not a long term solution. It's a temporary tool to help you learn. Once learned, let it go and trust yourself to implement it.

Calorie counting, food tracking, and other methods of documenting what you eat to be sure you were "good" that day can cause negative mindset patterns. It can lead to obsessing over every single bite and playing the undereating game, where you try to beat yourself today by being better (eating less) than yesterday. That's a recipe for disaster. No more games! NO MORE!

A better measure is to visualize your 80/20 (or 90/10). If 80+% of every day is healthy and clean, you're good. No stress. At some point, you may need to tweak specific things such as fewer carbs, or something like that, but for the scope of this book, we will stick with the basics. It's hard to get fat on veggies. Don't overthink it.

One more thought on calories and counting: The best way to keep your calories in check is to watch your portion sizes. It's not always what we eat. (Even though quality is King!) Sometimes, it's the amount we are eating. Fill up on veggies—they are magic! If you really want to up your nutrition game and get results, like now, bump up your veggie intake and watch the magic happen! There is no better, healthier food on the planet than fresh (preferably organic) vegetables. Eat them in salads, smoothies, soups, roasted, grilled, sautéed, or any other way you want. They are the pinnacle of healthy eating, but you knew that already.

When you add more veggies, you're adding more fiber and nutrients and you will automatically fill up faster with fewer calories. (Magic!) This is where portions can help. Aim for 50% of each meal to be from veggies (and some fruit, but veggies still reign supreme). Add some protein and healthy fat and you're golden. That is an ideal healthy meal in my mind. The veggies have carbs, so you're not eliminating carbs here, just filling up on foods with tons of nutrition benefits. Think of a big salad with avocado (healthy fat) and black beans (protein and complex carbs). Yum—that's my idea of a good time!

We won't get into specifics on carbs, grains, and all that fun stuff that seems to be so over complicated lately. Basically, the bottom line is you can get all the carb energy you need from fruit and veggies. You do not NEED grains and starches in a healthy diet. However, life without rice, potatoes, or corn chips once in a while is not a life I'm willing to live (at least not as of the moment I'm writing this book). You don't have to give up all carbs, but be aware that if you don't burn it off as energy, it is stored as fat. We tend to eat waaaaayyy more than we need. Cutting back on processed carbs like bread, pasta, muffins, pretzels, cereal, and even rice cakes, can make a big difference in how you look, and how you feel. Stick with complex, high fiber carbs (like veggies and fruit) and your body will thank you. I promise.

Your body on crack (I mean, sugar)

Speaking of carbs and simple, refined foods, let's dip into this topic a little further. I promised to keep this book straightforward and simple, so I hope you don't mind a little extra time spent digging into this one because it's important, like really important, and it's very often misunderstood. Bear with me as we go a little deeper on this one.

Let's tackle the topic of sugar, sweeteners, and simple carbs for a moment. Sugar has addictive qualities. Literally. You can be addicted to sugar.

All sugar. In any form. It's been shown in research to be more addictive than cocaine. It lights up all sorts of happy, pleasure centers in your brain, and you get a rush. It's just like a hit of an addictive substance (because it is). And it comes with the crash and cravings for more, just like any addictive substance. It's legit. It's not a joke, a weakness, or a choice.

Not everyone is as sensitive to it as others, kinda like alcohol. Some can handle it in moderation, or even large quantities, while others cannot have one sip without negative consequences and most likely a binge. That's the side I live on— the no moderation, binge crazy, super sensitive to sugar end of the spectrum. It's real. It could be what's preventing you from losing weight and feeling great. Not because you're weak and can't control yourself. Not because you need more willpower. Simply because it literally has a grip on you and you can't fight the urges and cravings of an addiction without awareness, strategies, and a plan.

Similarly, artificial sweeteners are not much better. Remember the whole quality and real food discussion? Artificial sweeteners are neither quality nor real. They are human-made chemicals that have no business being ingested as food.

Same with artificial anything for that matter: colors, flavors, preservatives, etc. We were not created to eat science experiments. We were created to eat the food provided by our Creator. It's really not complicated. The food industry, and the diet industry, has made it much more confusing than it needs to be.

One final note on sugar: Alcohol is sugar. If you choose to have alcohol as part of your 10-20% remember that it is a treat, so treat it like a dessert. If you have a drink, that is your treat for that meal (maybe for the day depending on your goals). Limit it. Pay attention to how you feel, your cravings, your energy, and your belly (bloated?) the next day. If you're stuck, or having a hard time with energy and cravings, eliminate alcohol for a while.

I personally don't drink—like ever. I know, I'm strange. So, I don't struggle with this one, but it comes up often with my clients, so I wanted to include it here for you. Even wine is a treat. You do not need it. It is "empty calories" (calories with little nutritional value), and it could be sabotaging your results.

Finally, as with all things, no diet plan, trainer, expert, or whatever knows you like you know yourself. You need to know what you can live without and what you just can't possibly even consider giving up. You will need to experiment with new foods. You will need to do things a little differently, and be patient with yourself as you learn and figure this stuff out. I do not have a one-size-fits-all solution that will work for everyone. It doesn't exist. I've never found a plan or diet I could follow 100%. I tweak and modify everything. At the moment, I eat a mostly vegan (I call it vegan-ish), gluten-free, and mostly sugar-free diet. It took time and many experiments to find what works for me, and it evolves over time.

It will take some trial and error for you too. But you're an intelligent person who is more than capable of figuring out how, and what, to eat in a way that is as healthy as possible without making this whole process overwhelming. You got this! Now go eat some veggies—green ones for bonus points!

REST

The next step in your journey to a healthier you, is to make sure you're getting enough sleep and rest. Yes, I said sleep AND rest. They are two different things and you need both.

I am not naive. I know how busy you are. You wouldn't be reading a book with simple, basic tips if you had all the time in the world to spend on fancy, advanced techniques or weekends away at retreats and spas. Hear me out: You cannot keep burning the candle at both ends and expect to feel amazing. It won't happen. You NEED downtime, and probably much more than you're getting currently.

Don't panic! You really don't need a life of luxury to get enough rest. (That would be nice, but probably not realistic.) You do need to be intentional about it. This is a crucial step that many people overlook. Not you. Not this time. You're learning the foundational steps to health and this is a big one. I'm begging you not to skim over this one!

Can you feel my intensity about this subject yet? I get a lot of push back on this step of the formula. For some reason, we are OK with being told to eat more veggies and get more exercise, but we're not OK with being told to get more rest. I don't get it. It's my favorite piece of the puzzle. It's part of the reward and enjoyment of a healthy life.

Stress could be sabotaging your weight goals

You have stress in your life, right? Yeah you do. We all do! It comes at us from all directions all day long. We live in a world of chronic stress and we think we have adapted to it. Most days we feel like we're handling things pretty well—maybe not great, but we're managing. That's not good enough. You're not managing. Not as well as you want. Not as well as I want for you.

If you're living in a chronic state of stress, constantly reacting, handling, and dealing with stress, even every day, seemingly insignificant stress, you're in a flight or fight mode way too often.

OK, you get it. We're all stressed out and full of stress hormones. So what? Maybe you like that feeling of the rush of a deadline or crossing things off your ridiculously long to-do list. Here's the problem with high stress levels: Stress messes you up! Stress can hinder weight loss, or even cause weight gain.

Yup, high stress and not enough sleep could be what's making you fat. For real. It might have nothing (or little) to do with what you eat and how much you exercise. Don't ignore those, but if you've tried everything else and you're still stuck, get more sleep!

Sleep is your BFF. Sleep reduces those stress hormones and allows the body to recover—from workouts, from life, from stress of all types.

What's your sleep number?

Well, just like everything else, that's an individual answer and there is not a one-size-fits-all answer. Here's what I've learned in my research and experience: Most adults need at least 7 hours. 7 hours minimum! And you thought 7 hours was a luxury, didn't you? If not, you're in the minority and one step closer to your goals than many.

Some adults require up to 9 hours to feel their best. 9 hours—like every night! Craziness, right? I know! But it's biology. Or physiology, or some other science-ology that you cannot change no matter how busy you are. Sleep, my friend. Lots of sleep.

Now be careful here: more than 9 hours tends to have the opposite effect. You'll wake up just as groggy and tired as if you had only a few hours. It's important to find your zone and stay in it consistently. How many hours would you sleep on vacation without an alarm clock? What's your natural sleep cycle? Aim for somewhere between 7 and 9 hours, and find the amount that is just right for you. This whole process is kind of like Goldilocks—you need to try it all and find what's right for you.

Do whatever it takes to get a solid night's sleep with as few interruptions as possible. There are many tips to help you actually sleep once your head hits the pillow. Google sleep habits or sleep hygiene for some help if you struggle to fall asleep or stay asleep. A dark, silent room with warm, comfy blankets works for me, but many do better with white noise and a cool room.

If you cannot get a solid stretch of at least 7 hours, it's not hopeless. Naps help. They're not ideal, but ultimately, sleep is sleep, and if napping is what it takes to get your hours in, then do what you gotta do my friend. You have permission to take a siesta!

Let's get back to the difference between sleep and rest. You know where I stand on sleep, as in actual shut-eye sleep. Now let's chat about rest.

The difference between sleep and rest

Let me back up and explain exactly what I mean by sleep and rest.

Sleep is essential for health. You know you get cranky and less than brilliant when you're sleep deprived. Remember the sleepless nights of new motherhood? Not so fun the next day.

Sleep is when your body does all sorts of awesome things to help you recover, reduce stress levels, and function well. It's super important for your brain, your weight loss, and your overall health.

Rest is an important part of a healthy life. Let's look at it from two angles: downtime (or chillax time) and rest from workouts, or the standard "Rest Day" approach.

Downtime, as in Netflix, hobbies, family game night, date night, or anything else that is pure enjoyment, is necessary. You need time for fun, for relaxation. Downtime is a lot like sleep in that each person requires different amounts to feel fulfilled. How much chill out time would you like to have on vacation? I'm talking an extended vacation beyond the first few days of catching up on your rest. When the novelty of being on vacation wears off and you can just breathe. What would that look like? Would you be lying on a beach or would you be exploring? That says a lot about your level of chillax-ness. (That's not a real word, but I think it could be.)

I'm not encouraging you to be a couch potato and spend all your free time resting. I am encouraging you to stop running yourself into the ground and enjoy some guilt free, unproductive, downtime on a regular basis. It's not exclusive to vacation mode.

Now let's talk about rest from a physical perspective. When you exercise, you cause stress in your body. This is a great example of how some stress can be good, as long as we rest and recover from it. Exercise is good stress. We need it. You need it, but it might not need to be as intense or as much as you think. Long, intense, hard workouts every day are a recipe for injury and burnout.

If (when) you work out consistently, the days you are not exercising are just as important as the ones you are. Working out while chronically sore and tired will not get you the results you want, nor will it allow your body to properly recover. That means sleep and rest. Muscles repair during sleep and rest. (I told you awesome things happen when you sleep.) As you get more fit, you will recover faster and may not need a rest day, but you still want to make sure you're not pushing through fatigue and soreness. Working smarter will get you further than pushing too hard.

Once again, this is not an invitation to lie around and do nothing because it's your Rest Day. Think of your workout days an intense activity and your non-workout days as active rest days. You can still be active, walking, hiking, playing, stretching, etc., without being intense.

In fact, low intensity movement (like walking) is a great Active Rest Day activity. A body in motion stays in motion. We're building momentum here with your healthy habits. Going from a day of challenging exercise to a day, or two, of lying around doing nothing (at least nothing physical) stops the momentum you've been building. Keep moving forward day by day, but take it easy and gentle some days. Not all workouts need to be challenging.

If anyone ever deserves a full-fledged, lie on the couch all day, 100% complete rest day, it is a marathoner (especially the charity runners who are everyday people and not elite athletes) the day after the race. How do I know? Because I've done it—twice. Not because I love to run, or because running comes naturally to me. In fact, it's the exact opposite. Running is hard. Marathons are one of the hardest things you can put your body through. And the pain is something I cannot adequately describe. Trust me when I tell you, the act of getting out of bed the next day is almost as hard as getting to the finish line!

Why am I telling you all this marathon stuff? No, I'm not going to suggest you run a marathon. In fact, I highly suggest against it, at least not until your fitness level is ready for it. (And it's totally cool with me if you never get to that point. Marathons are for the crazy people like me!) I'm telling you this little story because in 2016 I ran the Boston Marathon. Keep in mind that 'ran' is a relative term. I was in the waaaay back of the pack with the regular people, just trying to finish before the roads reopened!

I treated myself to lots of carbs and an Epsom salt soak that evening. I also treated myself to lots of snuggle time on the couch the next day. However,

I did get up at least every couple of hours to walk around (hobble and limp is more accurate), to keep my muscles from completely cramping up. I also taught a boot camp class that evening, in a gym that was on the second floor of a building without an elevator.

Don't be fooled, I did NOT work out that day, but I did force myself to tackle the stairs and walk around, and basically be actively resting. Lying around all day would have made the recovery process even longer. That's an example of active rest.

That's the difference between sleep, rest, and active rest. We need all of it. We need to find the right blend, the right amount of each. If you're an all-or-nothing, all-in type person, this part will be your biggest challenge. You're ready to know what to do, how to do it, and when to do it. You thought this book would be all about diet and exercise and you're ready for that. You may not be ready to be told to slow down. You thought you had to do more to lose weight and feel good. Maybe. That may be true, but in my experience, more often than not, sometimes you actually need to do less.

Finding your own kind of balance

Continuing to add more, and more, and more in an effort to feel better and be happier is the exact opposite of what you need to be doing, especially if you're sacrificing sleep to do it. You only have so much time and energy. We're working on increasing your energy, but it's still a finite resource.

I'm not a fan of using the word "balance" when referring to making time for everything on our plates. It makes me feel too fragile, like if one thing is out of whack, the balance point tips and everything comes crashing down. I like to think of everything in your life (your energy, your time, your priorities, your to-do lists, etc.) as sections of a pie chart or some sort of circle. It's like a cake. The cake is the complete thing with all of your stuff in it, all of it divided into different pieces. Some pieces can be cut into small bits (taking up less time and energy) and some pieces are cut into huge chunks (with extra frosting for me—at least back in the day), but ultimately, you're limited to the size of the cake. When it's gone, it's gone.

Now I want cake. Sorry about that. Maybe we should switch to a better, less tempting, analogy like the memory storage on your computer. The point is, it's a finite amount. Some things take up more space, and some take less, but they all have to fit within the limits. If not, you need to start deleting the things that don't matter to make room for the important stuff that is absolutely NOT deletable. That's what needs to happen in your life too, starting with making enough room for sleep and rest. Otherwise, you'll start slowing down and being less productive, just like a full storage device.

It's time to prioritize your health. That means opening up the time and energy it will take to make it happen. As talented and awesome as you are, even you cannot make something out of nothing (only God can do that). Be honest with yourself about your level of stress, and the many, many, many things you're trying to cram into the hard drive of your life. Something has to give before you crash for good. You can do anything, but you cannot do everything—at least not all at once.

You may be surprised at how much more productive you will be when you focus more on less.

FITNESS

Just like everything else we've covered so far, we're sticking with the basics when it comes to fitness. There are a lot of different theories, approaches, plans, and experts out there all saying slightly different things. There is a lot of room for variety and interpretation in fitness. I am going to keep it as simple for you as possible while also explaining some of the details, so you'll be able to decide where to start and what to do.

Just as veggies are King when it comes to food, form is King in fitness. Form refers to how your body moves. Are you doing the exercises as effectively and safely as possible? Is your back doing the work when your abs should be? Is your knee taking on too much pressure when your booty should be helping out more? Form is what helps prevent injury. Good form is going to get you results faster, because going through the motions with poor form will not get you great results. In fact, poor form will likely end up causing you an injury. Quality counts just as much here as it does with nutrition. Sloppy, unintentional movements are not effective. Good form and proper movement will help you be effective and safe.

It's hard to teach good form in a book—it's a visual thing for me. You can access form tutorials on my YouTube Channel and in the freebies on the book resource page (links in the appendix) to help get you started. Basically, you want your posture to be as tall as possible with all your joints lined up: ear over shoulder, shoulder over hip, hip over knee, knee over ankle. Keep the shoulders pulled down and back away from the ears, and keep the lower back in a natural curve.

There is more to it than that, but knowing that much will help you be more intentional in your movements. Working one-on-one with a trainer can help you identify where your form is off and how to correct it. If anything is painful (not simply uncomfortable), please stop. Something is not right if you feel pain. I do not believe in "no pain, no gain." Challenging, difficult, and uncomfortable? Yes. Pain? No. Pain usually begins with poor form. which is why it is vitally important that you be aware of how your body moves and how it could move better.

If you are unsure of your form and cannot figure out how to make it better, please reach out to me for a complimentary consultation. A quick conversation with a few simple techniques may be all you need to hit the ground running—or walking! Info on scheduling a call with me is in the appendix.

OK, now that your form is taken care of, let's get into some specifics. You probably want to know what type of exercise you should do, how often, and how long. Great questions. As with all things, everyone will be different. There are a lot of factors that help determine the best path for you. I'll go over the biggest, most effective tips to help you get started. Let's dive into them!

As far as what type of exercise to do, you do not need a fancy gym or expensive equipment to get fit. Honestly. I use very little equipment in my own workouts now. I teach group classes using no equipment, and it's a great workout. Body weight workouts at home can be very effective and challenging, when you know what to do and how to do it. (We're getting there. Hang on.) A little room to move around is really all you need.

As for what type of exercise to do, I believe in variety and effective exercises that not only help you look better, but actually help you move better, not just for your workout, but for life. When you train for balance, endurance, strength, flexibility, and power, you're more efficient in everything you do. You'll have a better chance at preventing falls and injuries. You'll be able to lift groceries, and children, without throwing your back out of whack.

Fitness is not just about burning calories. It's about being able to do the things I want (and need) to do without hurting myself. It's about being stronger and more capable of physical things than I ever thought possible. It's about building strong bones. It's about preventing the weight gain that has become the norm with age—you don't have to accept it. Fitness is the fountain of youth! When you train for fitness, instead of calorie burn, you help slow the aging process! You've heard stories of fit, healthy, active people well into their later years. It's possible.

That is why I am a strong advocate for a variety of exercises. If you do the same thing all the time, you get good at that one thing, but you don't strengthen all the other aspects of your physical health. You may end up with overuse injuries, burnout, or plateaus, not to mention boredom.

My signature style of training is called the 5S Fit method. It includes 5 S's: Stability (balance), Sweat (endurance), Strength, Stretch, and Smile. It's a foundational program that hits each of the most important steps to building solid fitness habits. I've learned over the years that if any one piece is missing, the results aren't as good and the commitment to stay consistent lessens. Variety and fun are the spice of life, and that's true in your fitness too! More info about 5S in the appendix.

Let's talk about cardio. Most people think all they need to do is jump on an elliptical machine and burn a few hundred calories and that meets their workout need for the day. Wrong! Any cardio machine is just that—cardio. Cardio is good for working your heart muscle (the most important muscle you have), so it's not bad. It's just not the whole picture. There are more effective ways to get the cardio benefit and work on other aspects of your fitness at the same time.

However, steady state cardio (long, slow cardio like a leisurely walk) is a great way to reduce stress. Low intensity cardio sessions are not designed to burn a lot of calories. A casual stroll or playing with your kids may get you to move your body, clear your head, lower your stress level, and they can be fun. Feel free to add it into your routine just for the pure enjoyment of it. But if you do not enjoy it, do not torture yourself with it for the sake of fitness. There are many more effective things you can try that you just might enjoy!

If you're not convinced to get off the elliptical yet, let me remind you that cardio burns calories (boring) while strength training burns calories *and* changes the shape of your body. (Yes, please!) If you want a tighter, leaner, stronger body that burns more calories 24/7, you need strength training. Don't be scared. You don't have to be a bodybuilder to get the benefits of strength training. You can use your own body to train. Ever try to do a push up? That takes strength and is a very effective exercise for strengthening your upper body and core, all while making you sweat a little, and getting your heart pumping. That's what I mean by effective. I'm all about multi-purpose exercises!

Effective exercises

Compound exercises, circuit training, and intervals are a few of my favorite ways to train. You will get the heart healthy cardio benefits along with muscle sculpting, body toning benefits of more intense training in less time.

A compound exercise is a movement that works multiple muscles at once. An example would be a lunge. Multiple leg muscles, glutes, core, and balance are all working while doing a lunge. A non-compound move would be a bicep curl. The primary muscle doing the work is the bicep. You can make a bicep curl harder by adding more weight or changing the pace, but that's still an isolated move. Remember, we are building your foundation here. Isolated and specific body part training comes later. You want effective things that have multiple benefits in less time. Trust me! You can make a bicep curl a compound move by adding a lunge with it, or by standing on one leg. Anytime more than one thing is happening at once, you're being more effective and efficient!

Circuit training is a method of stacking one exercise after another without rest in between. Instead of doing 3 sets of lunges in a row with a break between each set (for example: 12 lunges, rest, 12 more lunges, rest...), you add all the other movements in your routine for the day and do them back to back, with as little rest as possible between each. An example would be to do a set of squats followed by a set of push ups, followed by lunges, followed by a plank. When you finish one round of all of the exercises in your workout, you take a break and repeat as many times as you can, breaking between each round.

Finally, intervals are a time based method of intense training. You set a timer for a certain amount of time to do the exercise, followed by a time to rest (between each exercise). You go all out during the exercise time since you know you'll get a break as soon as it's over. It's short but it's really intense. This is the opposite of the slow, steady state we talked about before. You will be short of breath if you push hard enough. Push as hard as you can, as long as you can, and then rest just long enough to be ready to go again for another interval. An example would be sprints. You go really hard, pumping as fast as possible, barely able to catch your breath, and then when you can go no more you recover for as long as it takes to be ready to go again. You can apply intervals to strength training too. Do as many squats, as deeply, quickly, and powerfully as possible, until your muscles are shaking, burning, and ready to give up. Then recover for only as long as you need.

Sometimes, I combine all of these techniques. I'll choose compound movements planned in a circuit with several different exercises one after another, but I'll use a timer and make it an interval. Here's an example using a 40 second work cycle with a 20 second rest between exercises: lunge with bicep curl; squat with shoulder press; plank with leg lift.

Do you see how much more efficient that is compared to just peddling away on a cardio machine? Yes, it's more challenging. But it's also done faster and you'll feel amazing! There's nothing quite like the rush of pushing through challenging physical things and doing more than you thought you could. It's a rush! If you want to feel like a superstar, try some intense training.

One final note on intensity: it is YOUR level of intensity. Please do not try to keep up with anyone else. No comparisons here. Push to your level of intense, whatever than means for you.

Think of it as a scale of 1-10, where 1 is at rest and 10 is the most intense you can imagine. When you are interval training, you want to be at a level 7-10. It needs to be challenging. If you have any medical concerns, please take it slower and build up as you get stronger. In general, unless you are going for your stress-reducing, casual stroll, you want your workouts to be a challenge. That's where the magic happens. They don't always have to be intense, but they should push you to get a little uncomfortable.

Finally, have FUN! Do things you enjoy or find a way to make it enjoyable with a great instructor, motivating music, or with friends. Do your best to enjoy it! Make it something you look forward to. It's like being a kid on the playground again! You get to have play time whenever you want! It's an adult recess break! That's the Smile piece of my 5S method. It's just as important as the other parts. In fact, it may be the most important, because if you don't enjoy it, you won't keep coming back for more. Dance, sing, be silly. Anything that makes fitness fun is fair game!

Let me leave you with a few final thoughts: Fitness is about making progress. It's about being a little better tomorrow than today. However, you will have bad days. You will have setbacks. It's not a steady climb upwards. There are twists and turns along the way. Stay on course. Ride out the bumps in the road. Remember that it will never be perfect. As you get stronger, you'll keep pushing for more challenging things. It doesn't get easy, but it gets better. Keep focused on progress over perfection. All of this is supposed to make you happier and reduce your stress. Keep it simple and just keep pushing forward, one step at a time.

When all else fails, smile and fake it 'til you make it! Your body will believe what your mind thinks. Think like an athlete, and eventually you'll start to feel like an athlete. (I know that seems crazy, but stranger things have happened!)

I believe in you. It's time for *you* to believe in you and take action! You have all you need to get started. I'm here for you anytime you get stuck or need a little extra push. I'd love to hear from you. Please don't hesitate to contact me with questions, concerns, or to celebrate your success. I love celebrating with you!

Stay in touch at www.purplepenguinfitness.com or email me at support@purplepenguinfitness.com

Don't forget to get your free resources at www.fitdamentalsbook.com

ACTION PLAN

Read to get started and make some changes?

Here's a brief summary of some of the action steps covered in this book to help you get started:

- Start each morning with 1-2 large glasses of water. (Add a splash of lemon juice and/ or apple cider vinegar for extra benefits.)
- Drink approximately half your body weight in ounces of water each day.
- Eat food without nutrition labels (like produce) and foods with 5 ingredients or less.
- Eliminate High Fructose Corn Syrup, artificial sweeteners, and artificial colors.
- Fill up on veggies. At a minimum eat 3 servings of veggies each day.
- Allow 10% of your food to be treat foods,

but avoid foods you know you cannot eat in moderation. If you can't eat just one, then don't start.

- Get 7-9 hours of sleep each night!

- Schedule downtime to recharge each week.
- Schedule workouts. Have a plan and stick to it! 3 workouts per week to start.
- Sample workout without equipment using 30 second intervals (adapt the intervals as needed):

> 30 seconds of squats/ 30 seconds rest.
>
> 30 seconds of push ups/ 30 seconds rest.
>
> 30 seconds of standing 1 leg extensions (lift leg out straight to the side while .
>
> balancing on other leg)/ 30 second rest and repeat other side.
>
> 30 seconds plank/ 30 seconds rest.
>
> 30 seconds of Superman or flutter kicks/30 seconds rest.
>
> Total 6 minutes. Rest and repeat 1-4 times.

APPENDIX

These resources will be listed on www. fitdamentalsbook.com but you can also go directly to them from here.

Stay up to date on all things Purple Penguin Fitness at: www.purplepenguinfitness.com.

YouTube Channel: Search for Jenn Vazquez or direct link: http://bit.ly/PPFYT (case sensitive) .

Quiz to determine if you're really ready to make changes and stick with them: http://bit.ly/PPFreadyquiz.

My favorite home exercise toys, protein powder, and other must haves on Amazon: http://bit.ly/favesPPF.

If you're ready to get going and need a little push, I'd love to talk with you about how we can work together. No obligation. Set up a free consultation call here: www.bit.ly/calljenn.

Purple Penguin Fitness Fitdamentals Facebook® Group. Join the FB group with other Purple Penguins at www.tinyurl.com/ppfclub.

Find me on social media @jennvazquez17 (or Purple Penguin Fitness) on most platforms.

ABOUT THE AUTHOR

Jenn Vazquez is a personal trainer, fitness instructor, and weight loss coach. Basically, she helps women enjoy moving their bodies. She founded Purple Penguin Fitness to make fitness fun and accessible to women who are intimidated by the gym scene. Her motivation? Because she's been one of those women and has learned that fitness can, and should, be fun. She spent her early adult life as a hairstylist so, clearly, helping women feel good is important to her. She has been married to the love of her life since she was 19 (that's 23 years if you're counting) and they have two boys (young men) who light up her life. She also has an adopted daughter: a rescue dog named Lexi. Wife and mom are the most important titles she has. Marathoner, trainer, and author come close.

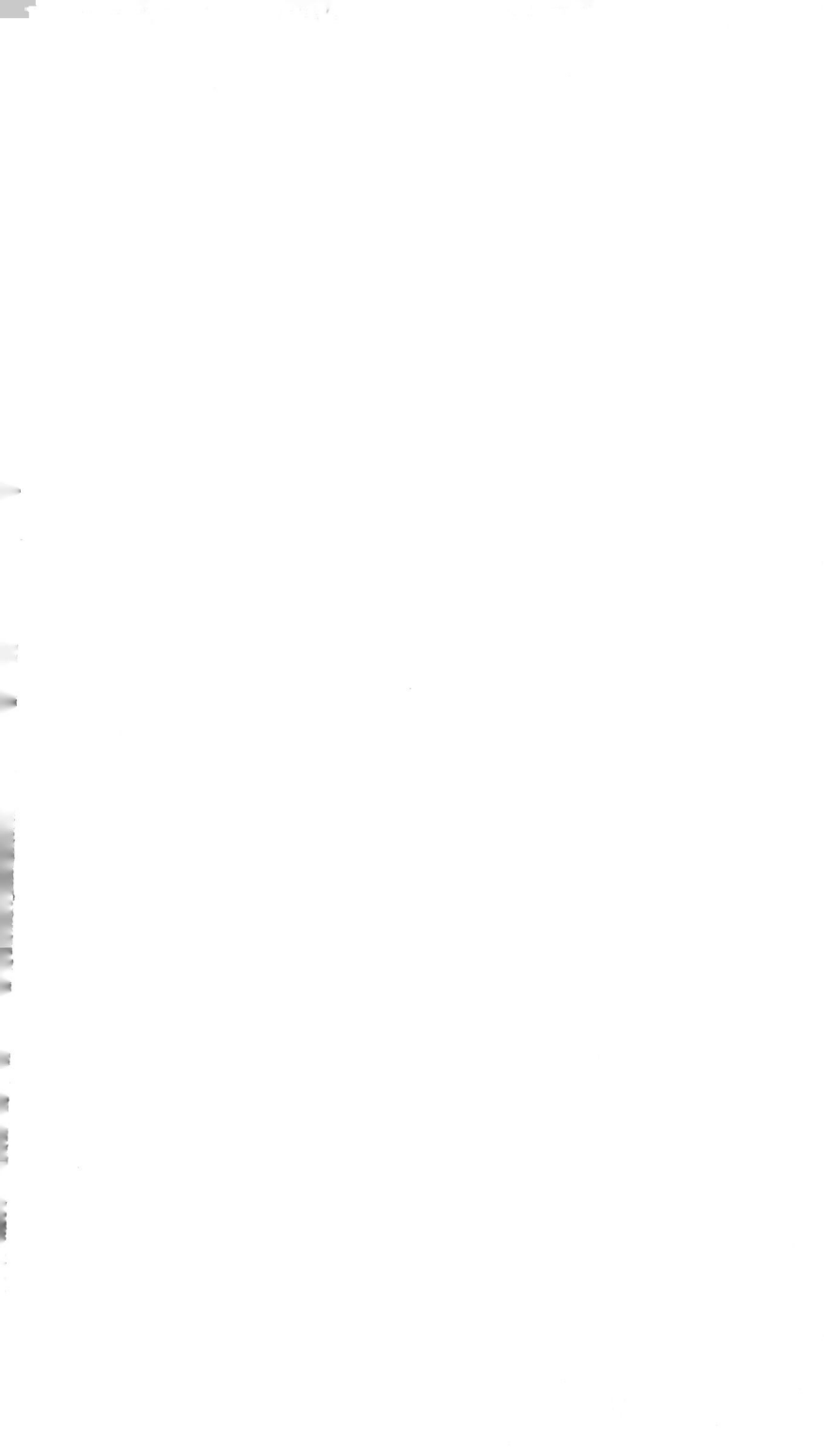

www.ingramcontent.com/pod-product-compliance
Lightning Source LLC
Chambersburg PA
CBHW050236270326
41914CB00034BA/1940/J